THIS BOOK

BELONGS TO

....

....

....

7 Home Remedies for Managing High Blood Pressure

There are several home remedies that can be used to help manage high blood pressure levels and improve heart health, including making changes to your diet and lifestyle.

What is high blood pressure?

Blood pressure is the force at which blood pumps from the heart into the arteries. A normal blood pressure reading is less than 120/80 millimeters of mercury (mm Hg).

When blood pressure is high, the blood moves through the arteries more forcefully. This puts increased pressure on the delicate tissues in the arteries and damages the blood vessels.

High blood pressure, or hypertension, affects about half of American adults, estimates the American College of Cardiology.

Known as a "silent killer," it usually doesn't cause symptoms until there's significant damage done to the heart. Without visible symptoms, most people are unaware that they have high blood pressure.

1. Get moving

Staying active is an important part of healthy living.

Along with helping lower blood pressure, regular physical activity benefits your mood, strength, and balance. It also decreases your risk of diabetes and other types of heart disease.

If you've been inactive for a while, talk with a doctor about a safe exercise routine. Start out slowly, then gradually pick up the pace and frequency of your workouts.

Not a fan of the gym? Take your workout outside. Go for a hike, jog, or swim and still reap the benefits. The most important thing is to get moving!

The American Heart Association (AHA) also recommends incorporating muscle strengthening activity at least 2 days per week. You can try lifting weights, doing pushups, or performing any other exercise that helps build lean muscle mass.

2. Follow the DASH diet

Following the Dietary Approaches to Stop Hypertension (DASH) diet can lower your systolic blood pressure by as much as 11 mm Hg. The DASH diet consists of:

- eating fruits, vegetables, and whole grains

- eating low fat dairy products, lean meats, fish, and nuts

- eliminating foods that are high in saturated fats, such as processed foods, high fat dairy products, and fatty meats

It also helps to cut back on desserts and sweetened beverages, such as soda and juice.

3. Limit salt

Reducing your sodium intake can be vital for lowering blood pressure.

In some people, when you eat too much sodium, your body starts to retain fluid. This results in a sharp rise in blood pressure.

The AHA recommends limiting your sodium intake to between 1,500 milligrams (mg) and 2,300 mg per day, which is a little over half a teaspoon of table salt.

To decrease sodium in your diet, try using herbs and spices to add flavor to foods in place of salt.

Processed foods also tend to be loaded with sodium. Be sure to always read food labels and choose low sodium alternatives when possible.

4. Maintain a moderate weight

Weight and blood pressure go hand in hand. For people with overweight or obesity, losing even just 5 to 10 pounds can help lower blood pressure levels.

In addition to reaching and maintaining a moderate weight, keeping tabs on your waistline is also critical for managing blood pressure. The extra fat around your waist, called visceral fat, may negatively affect heart health and could lead to serious health problems in the long run, including high blood pressure.

In general, men should keep their waist measurement to less than 40 inches while women should aim for less than 35 inches.

5. If you smoke, consider quitting

Each cigarette you smoke temporarily raises blood pressure for several minutes after you finish. If you smoke regularly, your blood pressure can stay elevated for extended periods of time.

People with high blood pressure who smoke are at greater risk for developing dangerously high blood pressure, heart attack, and stroke.

Even secondhand smoke can put you at increased risk for high blood pressure and heart disease.

Aside from providing numerous other health benefits, quitting smoking can help your blood pressure return to normal.

Visit our smoking cessation center to take steps to quit today.

6. Limit alcohol

Enjoying a glass of red wine with your dinner is perfectly fine. In fact, red wine might even be beneficial for heart health when consumed in moderation.

However, drinking excessive amounts of alcohol can lead to lots of health issues, including high blood pressure.

Excessive drinking can also reduce the effectiveness of certain blood pressure medications.

What does drinking in moderation mean? The AHA recommends that men limit their consumption to two alcoholic drinks per day. Women should limit their intake to one alcoholic drink per day.

One drink equals:

- 12 ounces of beer
- 4 ounces of wine
- 1.5 ounces of 80-proof liquor

7. Reduce stress

In today's fast-paced world that's filled with increasing demands, it can be hard to slow down and relax. However, it's important to step away from your daily responsibilities from time to time to help manage stress levels.

Stress can temporarily raise your blood pressure. Too much of it can keep your pressure up for extended periods of time.

It helps to identify the trigger for your stress. It may be your job, relationship, or finances. Once you know the source of your stress, you can try to find ways to fix the problem.

You can also take steps to relieve your stress in a healthy way. Try taking a few deep breaths, meditating, or practicing yoga.

The risks of high blood pressure

When left untreated, high blood pressure can lead to serious health complications, including stroke, heart attack, and kidney damage. Regular visits to a doctor can help you monitor and control your blood pressure.

A blood pressure reading of 130/80 mm Hg or above is considered high. If you've recently received a diagnosis of high blood pressure, a doctor can help determine the best course of treatment based on your needs.

Your treatment plan might include medication, lifestyle changes, or a combination of therapies. Taking the above steps can help bring your numbers down, too.

Staying active, decreasing salt intake, and making other dietary changes may lower blood pressure even more.

Frequently asked questions

What should be avoided in high blood pressure?

Several factors can contribute to high blood pressure, including inactivity, excessive alcohol intake, and a high sodium diet.

Staying active, moderating your alcohol intake, and limiting your consumption of processed foods and other high sodium ingredients may be beneficial.

Can drinking lots of water lower blood pressure?

Some research suggests that dehydration could contribute to high blood pressure levels by impairing the function of the blood vessels. Therefore, staying hydrated by drinking plenty of water throughout the day could be beneficial.

According to the Academy of Nutrition and Dietetics, men typically need around 13 cups of water per day while women require approximately 9 cups. However, this amount can vary depending on many factors, including your age, health status, and activity level.

How can I lower my blood pressure immediately?

There's no way to lower blood pressure levels immediately at home. Instead, you should develop a treatment plan with a doctor to reduce blood pressure levels in the long term, which may involve making changes to your diet, exercise routine, and lifestyle.

Takeaway

High blood pressure is a serious condition that can cause long lasting damage to the heart and blood vessels over time.

There are several home remedies that can help manage high blood pressure levels, including reducing your sodium intake, staying active, decreasing stress levels, and limiting your intake of alcohol.

If you have been diagnosed with high blood pressure, be sure to work with a healthcare professional to develop a treatment plan based on your needs.

High Blood Pressure Symptoms

High blood pressure

High blood pressure is often associated with few or no symptoms. Many people have it for years without knowing it.

However, just because high blood pressure is often symptomless doesn't mean it's harmless. In fact, uncontrolled high blood pressure, or hypertension, causes damage to your arteries, especially those in the kidneys and eyes. High blood pressure is also a risk factor for stroke, heart attack, and other cardiovascular problems.

High blood pressure is generally a chronic condition. There are two major categories of high blood pressure: secondary hypertension and primary hypertension. Most people have primary hypertension, otherwise known as essential hypertension.

- Secondary hypertension is high blood pressure that is the direct result of a separate health condition.

- Primary hypertension is high blood pressure that doesn't result from a specific cause. Instead, it develops gradually over time. Many such cases are attributed to hereditary factors.

Typically, the only way to know you have hypertension is to get your blood pressure tested.

Rare symptoms and emergency symptoms

Rarely, people with chronic high blood pressure might have symptoms such as:

- dull headaches

- dizzy spells

- nosebleeds

When symptoms do occur, it's usually only when blood pressure spikes suddenly and extremely enough to be considered a medical emergency. This is called a hypertensive crisis.

Hypertensive crisis is defined as a blood pressure reading of 180 milligrams of mercury (mm Hg) or above for the systolic pressure (first number) *or* 120 or above for the diastolic pressure (second number). It's often caused by skipping medications or secondary high blood pressure.

If you're checking your own blood pressure and get a reading that high, wait a few minutes and then check again to make sure the first reading was accurate. Other symptoms of a hypertensive crisis may include:

- severe headache or migraine

- severe anxiety

- chest pain

- vision changes

- shortness of breath

- nosebleed

After waiting a few minutes, if your second blood pressure reading is still 180 or above, don't wait to see whether your blood pressure comes down on its own. Call 911 or your local emergency services immediately.

Emergency hypertensive crisis can result in severe complications, including:

- fluid in the lungs
- brain swelling or bleeding
- a tear in the aorta, the body's main artery
- stroke
- seizures in pregnant women with eclampsia

High blood pressure during pregnancy

In some cases, high blood pressure can occur during pregnancy. There are several types of high blood pressure disorders in pregnancy. Causes may be due to a number of factors, including:

- obesity
- chronic high blood pressure
- diabetes
- kidney disease
- lupus
- in vitro fertilization (IVF) and other pregnancy-related assistance
- being a teen or being over 40 years of age
- carrying more than one child (e.g., twins)
- first-time pregnancy

If high blood pressure occurs during pregnancy after 20 weeks, a condition known as preeclampsia may develop. Severe preeclampsia can cause damage to the organs and brain, which can bring on life-threatening seizures known as eclampsia.

Signs and symptoms of preeclampsia include protein in urine samples, intense headaches, and vision changes. Other symptoms are abdominal pain and excessive swelling of the hands and feet.

High blood pressure during pregnancy can cause a premature birth or early detachment of the placenta. It may also require a cesarean delivery.

In most cases, the blood pressure will return to normal after giving birth.

Complications and risks of high blood pressure

Over time, untreated high blood pressure can cause heart disease and related complications such as heart attack, stroke, and heart failure.

Other potential problems are:

- vision loss
- kidney damage
- erectile dysfunction (ED)
- fluid buildup in the lungs
- memory loss

Treatment for high blood pressure

There are a number of treatments for high blood pressure, ranging from lifestyle changes to weight loss to medication. Doctors will determine the plan based on your level of high blood pressure and its cause.

Dietary changes

Healthy eating is an effective way to help lower high blood pressure, especially if it's only mildly elevated. It's often recommended to eat foods low in sodium and salt, and high in potassium.

The Dietary Approaches to Stop Hypertension (DASH) diet is one example of a food plan prescribed by doctors to keep blood pressure in order. The focus is on low-sodium and low-saturated fat foods such as fruits, vegetables, and whole grains.

Some heart-healthy foods include:

- apples, bananas, and oranges
- broccoli and carrots
- brown rice and whole-wheat pasta
- legumes
- fish rich in omega-3 fatty oils

Foods to limit are:

- foods and drinks high in sugar
- red meat
- fats and sweets

It's also suggested to not consume excess alcohol while trying to manage high blood pressure. Men should have no more than two drinks a day. Women should have no more than one drink.

Exercise

Physical activity is another important lifestyle change for managing high blood pressure. Doing aerobics and cardio for 30 minutes with a goal of five times a week is a simple way to add to a healthy heart routine. These exercises will get the blood pumping.

With good eating and exercise comes a healthy weight. Proper weight management helps lower cholesterol and high blood pressure. Other risks caused by being overweight are also decreased.

Another way to treat high blood pressure is by trying to manage and limit stress. Stress will raise blood pressure. Try different methods of stress relief such as exercise, meditation, or music.

Medication

There are a variety of medications that can be used to treat high blood pressure if lifestyle changes alone aren't helping. Many cases will require up to two different medications.

diuretics	Also called water or fluid pills, diuretics wash out excess fluid and sodium from the body. These are most often used with another pill.
beta-blockers	Beta-blockers slow the heartbeat. This helps less blood flow through the blood vessels.
calcium channel blockers	Calcium channel blockers relax the blood vessels by blocking calcium from going inside cells.
angiotensin-converting enzyme (ACE) inhibitors	ACE inhibitors block hormones that raise blood pressure.
alpha blockers and central acting agents	Alpha blockers relax blood vessels and block hormones that tighten the blood vessels. Central acting agents make the nervous system decrease nerve signals that narrow the blood vessels.

When to see your doctor for high blood pressure

Call your doctor if any of these treatments aren't working to lower high blood pressure. It can take up to two weeks for a new medication to have its full effect. No change in your blood pressure may mean another treatment is needed, or it can be the result of another problem occurring with the high blood pressure.

You should also call your doctor if you experience:

- blurry vision

- headaches

- fatigue

- nausea

- confusion

- shortness of breath

- chest pain

These can also be the symptoms of something else or a side effect of the medication. In this instance, another medicine may need to be prescribed to replace the one causing discomfort.

Outlook for high blood pressure

Once you have high blood pressure, you are expected to monitor and treat it for the rest of your life. There is a chance the high blood pressure returns to normal with lifestyle changes, but it's challenging. Both lifestyle changes and medicine are typically needed in order to maintain a goal blood pressure. Treatment will also greatly lower the chance of heart attack, stroke, and other heart disease-related complications.

With careful attention and proper monitoring, you can lead a healthy life.

What Are the Symptoms of High Blood Pressure in Women?

Blood pressure is the force of blood pushing against the inside lining of the arteries. High blood pressure, or hypertension, occurs when that force increases and stays higher than normal for a period. This condition can damage the blood vessels, heart, brain, and other organs.

Hypertension is often considered a men's health problem, but that's a myth. The American Heart Association reports that about half of people with high blood pressure are women. High blood pressure impacts 1 in 3 Americans in their 40s, 50s, and 60s. Gender doesn't usually impact the risk greatly, but the onset of menopause slightly raises the risk of developing high blood pressure.

Language matters

Most of the sources used in this article use "men" and "women" to indicate sex and can be assumed to have primarily cisgender participants. But like most conditions, sex and assigned gender are not the most likely indicator of high blood pressure.

Your doctor can better help you understand how your specific circumstances will translate into diagnosis, symptoms, and treatment for high blood pressure.

Symptoms of high blood pressure in women

High blood pressure doesn't always cause symptoms. In fact, it's sometimes referred to as a "silent condition" because most people with high blood pressure have no symptoms at all.

Often, symptoms don't appear at all until someone has had high blood pressure for years and the condition has become severe, but even people with severe high blood pressure might have no symptoms at all.

When symptoms do occur, they look the same in everyone and might include:

- skin flushing

- red spots in front of the eyes

- dizziness

But these symptoms only occur once elevated blood pressure has caused the damaged blood vessels to break. The only real sign of high blood pressure is getting consistently high blood pressure readings. That's why it's important to have your blood pressure checked at least once a year.

Symptoms of high blood pressure in elderly women

There's no change to the symptoms of high blood pressure as a person ages. Although cis women who are past menopause are at higher risk for high blood pressure, they're still unlikely to experience any symptoms at all. High blood pressure is still a silent condition in older women.

If any symptoms do occur, they'll be likely to be flushing, red spots in front of the eyes, and dizziness. But the best way for older women to monitor their blood pressure is to keep track of their blood pressure numbers and have conversations about their blood pressure with their healthcare professional.

The overall risk for high blood pressure goes up as everyone ages, regardless of sex or gender.

High blood pressure in transgender women

While less research has been done on high blood pressure within transgender women, there are some indications that transgender individuals are overall more likely to experience higher rates of cardiovascular diseases — possibly due to the role of stress in the development of these diseases.

But a large study in 2021 showed that stage 2 hypertension decreased by 47 percent within 4 months of gender-affirming hormone therapy.

Complications of high blood pressure

Without proper diagnosis, you may not know that your blood pressure is increasing. Uncontrolled high blood pressure can lead to damage to the blood vessels of various organs. This can cause serious health problems, like:

- stroke
- kidney failure
- heart attacks
- weakened or thickened blood vessels in your kidneys
- dementia
- vision problems

There's also evidence to suggest that high blood pressure might put you at a higher risk of becoming severely ill if you contract COVID-19.

Understanding preeclampsia

If you're pregnant, high blood pressure can be especially dangerous for both you and your baby. Both those who have preexisting high blood pressure and those without may experience pregnancy-induced hypertension — which is related to the more serious condition called preeclampsia.

Preeclampsia affects around 5 percent of pregnancies and is one of the leading causes of both maternal and infant mortality.

Generally, preeclampsia develops during the 20th week of pregnancy, but it can occur earlier in rare cases. It can also sometimes occur during postpartum. The symptoms include high blood pressure, headaches, possible liver or kidney problems, and sometimes sudden weight gain and swelling.

Fortunately, It's usually a manageable complication. It typically disappears within 2 months after the baby is born. The following characteristics raise your risk for preeclampsia:

- being a teenager

- being over 40

- having multiple pregnancies

- obesity

- a history of hypertension or kidney problems

When to see your doctor

The best way to find out if you have hypertension is by checking your blood pressure. This can be done at the doctor's office, at home with a blood pressure monitor, or even by using a public blood pressure monitor, like those found in shopping malls and pharmacies.

You should know your usual blood pressure. Then you can seek further evaluation from your healthcare professional if you see a significant increase in this number the next time your blood pressure is checked.

If you have experienced any possible symptoms mentioned above, it's important to tell your doctor right away. Symptoms very rarely occur with high blood pressure and could be a sign your blood pressure has been high for a long time.

Gender bias in medical diagnosis

The first step to getting the care and treatment you need is getting diagnosed. Unfortunately, this isn't always an easy process. It can take multiple appointments, tests, and even visits to many doctors before you have answers.

For women, this process can have additional frustrations. Studies have shown that gender biases in medicine can lead to delays in care, incorrect diagnoses, and other serious concerns for women.

In conditions more often thought of men's health conditions, such as high blood pressure, this can play an even bigger role. Doctors might not be looking for these conditions in women or might not be aware of how they present in women.

That's why it's important to know your own blood pressure numbers and advocate for yourself.

Preventing high blood pressure

Expert advice for preventing high blood pressure is the same for everyone:

- Exercise about 30 to 45 minutes per day, 5 days a week.

- Eat a diet that's moderate in calories and low in saturated fats.

- Stay current with your doctors' appointments.

Talk with your doctor about your risk for high blood pressure. Your doctor can let you know the best ways to keep your blood pressure in the normal range and your heart healthy.

Takeaway

High blood pressure is often thought of as a men's health concern, but that's not the case. High blood pressure can impact anyone, and gender doesn't increase or decrease your risk.

High blood pressure often has no symptoms at all and is thought of as a "silent condition." This is true for everyone, regardless of age or gender. But that doesn't mean it's not serious. If left untreated, high blood pressure can lead to strokes, heart attack, dementia, kidney failure, and more. That's why it's important to have your blood pressure checked at least once a year.

Table of Contents

INTRODUCTION

R esearch shows that about 70% adults in the United Sates are overweight or obese and about 30% of U.S adults have high blood pressure or hypertension. According to the WHO (World Health Organization), hypertension is a severe medical condition that significantly increases the risks of heart, brain, kidney and other illnesses.

One of the low moments in a person's life is when he or she has been diagnosed with high blood pressure, otherwise known as hypertension. This health condition can put a strain on a person's emotional, psychological, social and economic wellbeing.

Some immediate causes of hypertension are often not known since a number of individuals suffer this ailment due to their family history or blood line. While others are predisposed to high blood pressure due to some unhealthy habits formed over time such as excessive use of alcohol, lack of exercises or a sedentary lifestyle and the kinds of diet they eat. It is also a known fact that a person's likelihood f developing hypertension increases with the aging process.

Uncontrolled hypertension can result to dangerous health conditions like heart attack, kidney failure and stroke. Hence, it is advised to pay close attention to this particular ailment.

Having said all that, it is not all bad news, as hypertension can be controlled through understanding certain secrets. The good news I have for you is that you don't have to die of hypertension. As I write this book, I can assure you that I have a father who has lived with hypertension and has made it to 83 years old today!

Follow the simply secrets revealed in this book to help you understand better high blood pressure, it's causes and the ways of reversing it.

In this book, you will learn simply secrets about what causes your blood pressure to rise. I will take you through a journey to better understand hypertension, what causes it and simply routines that you will follow to help you reduce or lower your high blood pressure successfully.

CHAPTER ONE

What Is Hypertension?

igh blood pressure is another term for hypertension and it happens when your body has developed a lot of obstruction in your arteries, so pumping blood all through your body turns out to be very troublesome. This influences how hard your heart needs to function when it pumps blood. By working harder, your heart becomes stressed and won't work at its optimum limit.

Over the long haul, hypertension can truly influence your wellbeing by possibly causing coronary diseases, stroke and congestive cardiovascular breakdown among numerous different issues. Having a weak heart can likewise expose you up to serious vulnerabilities later as you advance in age.

It is not all bad news, notwithstanding, in the event that you are experiencing hypertension. Hypertension is profoundly treatable. A sound eating regimen, sleeping soundly, and exercise can all further ameliorate states of hypertension. Getting your blood pressure checked routinely can likewise assist with catching symptoms of other more extreme issues earlier.

Understanding Blood Pressure Readings

The machine used for measuring your blood pressure is known as a sphygmomanometer or blood pressure monitor. Some health specialists refer to them as blood pressure gauge. It is an instrument used to measure blood pressure and it is made up of an inflatable cuff to collapse and then release the artery under the cuff in a controlled manner. It also contains a mercury manometer that indicates the pressure. Manual sphygmomanometers are usually used in conjunction with a stethoscope when using the auscultatory technique. However, today, there are lots of electronic or digital (or automatic) sphygmomanometer that can be purchased off-shelf any pharmaceutical store.

In a manual method of blood pressure measurement, the doctor or nurse places a stethoscope over the main artery in your upper arm also known as the brachial artery, and listens to the blood flow. The cuff will be inflated with a little hand pump. As the cuff inflates, it is filled with air and it squeezes your arm. The blood flow in through your artery ceases momentarily. He or she then releases a valve on the hand pump to gradually release the air in the cuff and restore blood flow. He or she will continue to listen your blood flow, pulse and then record your blood pressure. The results of your blood pressure is indicated in millimeters of mercury (mm Hg) and the measurement has two numbers that look like a mathematical fraction. The numerator number (systolic) is the force of the blood flow when your heart muscle contracts, pumping blood. The denominator number (diastolic) is the pressure measured between heartbeats.

What Is Systolic Pressure?

Blood pressure is indicated via two numbers. The first number, which is usually at the top is called the systolic pressure. This number measures the pressure in your arteries when your heart beats. When your heart beats, it pumps and circulates blood through your arteries to the rest of your body. That force creates pressure on those blood vessels and that pressure is your systolic blood pressure.

What Is Diastolic Pressure?

The second number which is usually the denominator (number under the first one), called diastolic blood pressure. It indicates the pressure in your arteries when your heart relaxes between the beats.

What Is Normal Blood Pressure?

A blood pressure is composed this way: 120/80. It is read as "120 over 80." The top number is known as the systolic, and base number is known as the diastolic. The limits are:

- Normal: Under 120 over 80 (120/80)

- Raised: 120-129/under 80

- Stage 1 hypertension: 130-139/80-89

- Stage 2 hypertension: above 140 or greater than /90

- Hypertension emergency: higher than 180/higher than 120 - - See a specialist immediately

Assuming your blood pressure is over the normal range, discuss with your doctor about how to bring it down.

CHAPTER TWO

What Are The Causes Of Hypertension?

Blood pressure is the proportion of the force of blood pushing against the blood vessels. The heart pumps blood into blood vessels, which convey the blood all through the body. High Blood Pressure, also known as called hypertension, is risky on the grounds that it makes the heart work harder to pump blood out to the body and contributes to hardening of the supply arteries, or atherosclerosis, to stroke, kidney disease, and to cardiovascular failure.

The specific reasons for hypertension are not known, yet a few things might assume contribute, such as listed below.

Smoking

It had been medically proven with overwhelming evidence backing it, that cigarette smoking causes adverse cardiovascular events and acts collaboratively with hypertension and dyslipidemia to increase the risk of coronary heart disease. Smoking is known to cause a severe increase in blood pressure and heart rate and it had been discovered to be linked with uncontrollable hypertension.

Being Overweight Or Obese

Obesity is a major public health challenge globally and it is inseparably connected to adverse cardiovascular diseases. The correlation between excess corpulence and aggravated high blood pressure is well known. It is estimated that obesity contributed to over 70% of cases of primary hypertension.

About 70% adults in the United Sates are overweight or obese and about 30% of U.S adults have high blood pressure or hypertension. When you are overweight or obese, your heart works harder to pump blood through your body arteries. Those extra efforts put extra pressure on your arteries. Then your arteries counter this flow of blood resulting in a rise of your blood pressure. Obesity is a word used to define people who have a body mass index (BMI) of over 30 and it constitutes a major risk factor for high blood pressure.

Lack Of Physical Exercise

A consistent lifestyle marked with inactivity, especially a sedentary lifestyle can lead to high blood pressure. Poor lifestyle routine, such as a lack of exercise, can lead to high blood pressure. Working in certain professions where your job requires you to sit for long periods of time while working, such as being a virtual assistant or customer service agent can expose you to risks of developing hypertension. The less active you get, the less fit you become and have a 30-50 percent chance of developing high blood pressure. Since you are you exercising, your heart is not built strong leading to a weak heart that could find it more difficult pumping blood through the arteries of your body.

A Lot Of Salt In The Meal

How does salt aggravate blood pressure? When you consume a lot of salt, which contains sodium, your body tends to retain extra water it uses to cleanse or get rid of the salt from your body. That extra water which your body retains exerts stress on your heart and blood vessels. In certain individuals, this may result in heightened blood pressure.

A Lot Of Alcohol Consumption (More Than 1 To 2 Drinks Each Day)

Consuming a lot of alcohol can increase your blood pressure to dangerous levels. Taking more than three drinks in a sitting can temporarily shoot up your blood pressure. However, a continuous and sustained binge drinking can result in persistent or chronic increases in your blood pressure. It might be very helpful for you to understand the definitions of excessive alcohol intake.

Binge drinking is described as more than four drink within a two-hour timeframe for women and more than five drink within the same timeframe for men. Moderate alcohol consumption will be having at most one drink per day for women and two for men.

Heavy drinking constitutes more than three drinks per day for women and more than four drinks for men. Heavy drinks who reduce alcohol intake to moderate level can lower their systolic blood pressure number by up to 5.5 millimeters of mercury (mm Hg) while decreasing their diastolic pressure number by up to 4 mm Hg.

Stress

Your body tends to secrete a rush of hormones when you find yourself in a stressful situation. Then these hormones momentarily cause spikes in your blood pressure by triggering your heart to beat faster than normal and your blood vessels narrow, leading to an increase in blood pressure. There is no evidence that stress alone can lead to chronic high blood pressure. However, responding to stress in unhealthy ways can increase you risk of hypertension, heart failure and strokes.

Age

The probability of having high blood pressure heightens are one gets older, most especially in cases of isolated systolic hypertension. Increases in blood pressure (BP) as a result of aging, is seen as a universal phenomenon of human aging. For Westerners who are over 40 years, their systolic pressure increases approximately 7 mm Hg per decade. Studies have shown that a positive correlation exists between high blood pressure and advancing in age, by up to circa 140 mmHg in the eight decades.

As an individual ages his or her vascular system changes. The vascular system is composed of the heart and blood vessels. Within the blood vessels there is a reduction in the elastic tissue in his or her arteries, causing them to become inelastic and less malleable. This results in heightened blood pressure.

Aging brings about physiological changes which further leads to an increase in systolic blood pressure; a rise in mean arterial pressure, a rise in pulse pressure and a reduction in the ability to respond quickly to sudden hemodynamic changes. The increase in blood pressure associated with aging is usually related to arterial changes.

Hereditary Factors

Blood relations tend to share a lot of similar or the same genetic composition that can put a person at risk of developing high blood pressure, coronary diseases or stroke. Genes subtly contribute to predisposing an individual to high blood pressure, heart disease and similar conditions. Nevertheless, is it also possible that people with a family history (or genealogy) of high blood pressure partake in familiar habitats or environs or surroundings and other likely factors that could heighten their risk factors. Genes are components of heredity that are transmitted from parents to their offspring. Relative also share common lifestyles such as food or diet, exercise and smoking that could trigger risk. Often, hypertension tends to run in families such that persons whose parents suffer hypertension have a heightened risk of developing the condition, especially when both parents are affected.

Blood pressure (BP) is also a traditionally complicated genetic trait with heritability estimates about 30 - 50%.

Chronic Kidney Disease

The kidneys contribute in keeping your blood pressure within a healthy limit. Weakened kidneys are less capable of helping you regulate blood pressure. Your kidneys filter waste and sodium using tiny gauze called glomeruli that can sometimes become swollen. If the swollen glomeruli do not work effectively, it can lead you to developing high blood pressure.

Adrenal And Thyroid Disorders (Endocrine Connection)

The endocrine system is a chain of glands that secrete hormones that the body utilizes for a wide range of functions, including the regulation of blood pressure. When the adrenal glands produce excess aldosterone, cortisol, or hormones similar to adrenaline, it can cause high blood pressure. High blood pressure can also result from an underactive thyroid gland(hypothyroidism) or an overactive thyroid gland(hyperthyroidism). Often, the pituitary glands are the cause of the problems in the adrenal glands. For instance, if the pituitary gland transmits excessive signal to the adrenal glands or thyroid gland, this can cause a rise in blood pressure. Also, when the parathyroid glands release too much parathyroid hormone, this leads to heightened blood pressure. In the case of obese individuals, high blood pressure may be due partially to increased insulin levels and insulin resistance. Insulin is created in the pancreas.

Sleep Apnea

Sleep apnea causes a constriction to your airway during sleep. This leads to disrupted breathing and reduced air intake. In the case of obstructive sleep apnea, the issue begins in the throat muscles. Central sleep apnea, however, is as a result of a problem with the brain signals that help regulate breathing. A person might suffer both forms of sleep apnea and this condition is connected to high blood pressure.

Types Of Hypertension

Essential Hypertension (Aka Primary Hypertension)

In as much as 95% of hypertension cases in the U.S., the fundamental reason can't be found. This sort of hypertension is called essential hypertension or primary hypertension.

Even though essential hypertension remains fairly puzzling, it has been connected to specific risk factors. Hypertension will in general run in families and is bound to influence men than women. Age and race also contribute a part. In the US, blacks are two times as probable as whites to have hypertension, although the gap begins to close around age 44. After age 65, black women have the most significant frequency of hypertension.

Essential hypertension is also incredibly impacted by diet and lifestyle. The correlation between salt and hypertension is very significant. Individuals living on the northern islands of Japan eat more salt per capita than any other person on the planet and have the most noteworthy occurrence of essential hypertension.

The vast majority of people with hypertension are "salt sensitive," implying that anything over the minimal body requirement for salt is a lot for them and increase their blood pressure. Different elements that can raise the risk of having essential hypertension include obesity; diabetes; stress; inadequate intake of potassium, calcium, and magnesium; absence of physical exercise; and chronic alcohol consumption.

Secondary Hypertension

Whenever an immediate cause for hypertension can be isolated, the condition is known as secondary hypertension. Among the known factors for secondary hypertension, kidney disease is the most significant. Hypertension can likewise be triggered by cancers or different anomalies that cause the adrenal organs (little organs that sit on the kidneys) to discharge excessive measures of the hormones that raise blood pressure. Contraception pills - explicitly those containing estrogen - and pregnancy boost blood pressure, as could drugs that at any point choke the blood vessels.

Who Is More Likely To Develop Hypertension?

- Individuals with relatives who have hypertension

- Smokers

- African-Americans

- Pregnant women

- Women who take anti-conception medication pills

- Individuals beyond 35 years old

- Individuals who are overweight or obese

- Individuals who are not active

- Individuals who drink alcohol excessively

- Individuals who eat large amounts of greasy foods containing excess salt

- Individuals who suffer sleep apnea

CHAPTER THREE

Symptom Of High Blood Pressure

Once in a while, individuals with chronic hypertension could have symptoms like,

- dull headaches

- bleary eyed spells

- nosebleeds

At the point when such symptoms occur, it is typically just when blood pressure spikes out of nowhere and incredibly enough to be viewed as a health-related crisis. This is situation is known as a hypertensive emergency.

Hypertensive emergency is characterized as a blood pressure reading of 180 milligrams of mercury (mm Hg) or above for the systolic pressure (first number) or 120 or above for the diastolic pressure (second number). It is frequently caused by skipping medications or secondary hypertension.

Assuming you are checking your own blood pressure and get a reading that high, wait by a couple of minutes and then check again to ensure the first reading was precise. Different symptoms of a hypertensive emergency might include:

- serious migraine or headache

- extreme tension (or anxiety)

- chest pain

- vision changes

- windedness (or difficulty breathing)

- nosebleed

After waiting for a couple of minutes, assuming that your subsequent blood pressure reading is as still 180 or above, don't wait to see whether your blood pressure will decrease. Call 911 or your local emergency services immediately.

Emergency hypertensive crisis can bring about extreme complications, including:

- fluid in the lungs

- brain swelling or bleeding

- a cut in the aorta, the body's principal artery

- stroke

- seizures in pregnant ladies with eclampsia

Hypertension During Pregnancy

In rare cases, hypertension can occur during pregnancy. There are a few types of hypertension issues in pregnancy. Causes might be due to various factors, including:

- obesity

- chronic hypertension

- diabetes

- kidney illness

- lupus

- in vitro treatment (IVF) and other pregnancy-related help

- being a teenager or being over 40 years old

- carrying multiple children (e.g., twins)

- first-time pregnancy

Assuming that hypertension occurs during pregnancy after 20 weeks, a condition known as toxemia might develop. Serious toxemia can harm the organs and brain, which can cause life-threatening seizures known as eclampsia.

Some signs and symptoms toxemia or pre-eclampsia include protein in urine tests, serious migraines, and vision changes. Other symptoms are stomach pain and excessive swelling of the hands and feet.

Hypertension during pregnancy can cause a pre-mature birth or early detachment of the placenta. It might likewise require a surgical delivery.

Most of the time, the blood pressure will get back to normal after giving birth to a child.

CHAPTER FOUR

Reversing Hypertension By Adjusting Your Diet

By starting a couple of new food habits, such as counting calories and monitoring food quantities, you might be able to bring down your blood pressure and reduce the drugs you require to control hypertension. This is how you do it.

Monitor What You Eat

Certain individuals do not know the amount of calories that they eat and drink every day. They often misjudge the amount they eat and wonder why they cannot get more fit.

Recording the food you eat, including the quantities, can allow you to see reality with regards to your food intake. You can then begin scaling back - - diminishing calories and portions - to get leaner and control your blood pressure.

You should also be wary of your alcohol consumption. Alcohol is a known trigger for increased blood pressure.

Stay Away From Salt (Sodium)

A high-sodium diet increases blood pressure in many individuals. As a matter of fact, the less sodium you eat, the better blood pressure control you could achieve.

Experts recommend getting under 2,500 milligrams (mg) of sodium every day, except if you have hypertension or you are at risk (in the case that you have diabetes or kidney disease, or are an African American). In that case, you are advised to eat 1,500 milligrams of salt a day. That is under a teaspoon from every one of your meals and snacks.

To bring down the sodium in your eating regimen, attempt these ideas:

• Utilize a food journal to monitor the salt in the food varieties you eat.

• Break the cycle of habitually reaching out for your salt shaker. Table salt is around 40% sodium, as per the standard regulation. Hence, try not to add salt to your food once you begin to eat at the table.

• Read the labels while shopping. Search for lower-sodium grains, wafers, pasta sauces, canned vegetables, or any food varieties with low-salt options.

o Select foods that have 5% or less of the "Daily Value" of sodium.

o Avoid foods that have 20% or all the more Daily Value of sodium.

• Eat less of processed, canned, and packaged foods. Packaged, processed food varieties contribute to the vast amounts of the sodium in individuals' eating regimens. Assuming that you prepare your own food, you can control what is in it.

• At cafés, get some nutritional information about salt added to food. Many chefs will skip or scale back on salt if you inquire.

• Assuming your eatery posts the nutrition facts for its dishes, determine how much sodium is in a serving. There might be lower-sodium choices on the menu.

• Utilize salt-free salt flavors or seasonings.

• Assuming that you want to use salt while cooking, add it toward the end. You will have to add less.

Know What To Eat

Potassium, magnesium, and fiber, then again, may assist with controlling hypertension. Fruits and vegetables are high in potassium, magnesium, and fiber, and they are low in sodium. Stick to whole fruits and vegetables. Juice is less useful, since the fiber is eliminated. Additionally, nuts, seeds, vegetables, lean meats, and poultry are great sources of magnesium.

To increase the measures of normal potassium, magnesium, and fiber you take in, select from the following:

- apples

- apricots

- bananas

- beet greens

- broccoli

- carrots

- collards

- green beans

- dates

- grapes

- green peas

- kale

- lima beans

- mangoes

- melons

- oranges

- peaches

- pineapples

- potatoes

- raisins

- spinach

- squash

- strawberries

- yams

- tangerines

- tomatoes

- fish

- yogurt (without fat)

What Is The D.A.S.H. Diet?

DASH simply means Dietary Approaches to Stop Hypertension. The DASH diet is a smart dieting plan intended to help treat or forestall high blood pressure (hypertension).

The DASH diet includes food varieties that are high in potassium, calcium and magnesium. These supplements (or nutrients) assist with controlling blood pressure. This eating regimen limits food sources that are high in sodium, immersed fat and added sugars.

Studies have shown that the DASH diet can bring down blood pressure in just fourteen days. The eating regimen can likewise bring down low-density lipoprotein (LDL or "bad") cholesterol levels in the blood. Hypertension and high LDL cholesterol levels are two significant risk factors for coronary illness and stroke.

DASH Diet And Sodium

The DASH diet is lower in sodium than a normal American eating regimen, which can incorporate an astounding 3,400 milligrams (mg) of sodium or more daily.

The standard DASH diet limits sodium to 2,300 mg daily. It meets the recommendations from the Dietary Guidelines for Americans to keep everyday sodium intake to under 2,300 mg daily. That is generally how much sodium in 1 teaspoon of table salt.

A lower sodium adaptation of DASH limits sodium to 1,500 mg daily. You can pick the adaptation of the eating routine that meets your wellbeing needs. In the event that you do not know what sodium level is ideal for you, discuss with your primary care physician.

DASH Diet: What To Eat

The DASH diet is an adaptable and adjustable eating plan that makes a heart-healthy dieting style for a lifetime. It is not difficult to follow using food varieties found at your supermarket or grocery store.

The DASH diet is also rich in vegetables, fruits and whole grains. It incorporates no- fat or low-fat dairy items, fish, poultry, beans and nuts. It limits food sources that are high in saturated fat, like greasy meats and full-fat dairy products.

While following DASH, it is vital to pick food sources that are:

•	Contain lots of in potassium, calcium, magnesium, fiber and protein

•	Low in saturated fat

•	Low in sodium

Dietary Approaches to Stop Hypertension (DASH) is an eating plan rich in natural products, vegetables, whole grains, fish, poultry, nuts, vegetables, and low-fat dairy. These food varieties are high in key supplements like potassium, magnesium, calcium, fiber, and protein.

The DASH diet can bring down blood since it has less salt and sugar than the typical American eating regimen. The DASH diet removes pastries, improved refreshments, fats, red meat, and processed meats.

Women who followed the DASH diet for protracted periods reduced their risks of coronary artery disease and stroke.

To begin the DASH diet, follow these recommendations (in light of 2,000 calories every day):

•	Grains: 7-8 day to day servings (serving sizes: 1 cut of bread, 1/2 cup cooked rice or pasta, 1-ounce dry cereal)

•	Vegetables: 4-5 everyday servings (1 cup crude salad greens, 1/2 cup cooked vegetable)

•	Fruits: 4-5 day to day servings (1 medium fruit, 1/2 cup new or frozen organic fruit, 1/4 cup dried fruit, 6 ounces fruit juice)

•	Low-fat or fat-free dairy items: 2-3 day to day servings (8 ounces milk, 1 cup yogurt, 1.5 ounces cheddar or cheeses)

•	Lean meat, poultry, and fish: 2 or less servings daily (3 ounces cooked meat, poultry, or fish)

•	Nuts, seeds, and vegetables: 4-5 servings each week (1/3 cup nuts, 2 tablespoons seeds, 1/2 cup cooked dry beans or peas)

•	Fats and oils: 2-3 day to day servings (1 teaspoon vegetable oil or delicate margarine, 1 tablespoon low-fat mayonnaise, 2 tablespoons light plate of salad dressing)

•	Desserts: under 5 servings each week. (1 tablespoon sugar, jam, or jam)

Ask your primary care physician or a dietitian to assist you with beginning the DASH diet. They can show you the number of calories you need every day to keep up with or get to a healthy weight. And afterward they can assist you with arranging meals with food sources you love that meet the DASH diet guidelines.

Different Ingredients To Stay Away From

You definitely realize how salt can slip into a ton of packaged food varieties. Yet, it is not by any means the only thing to watch while you are monitoring your blood pressure.

Sugar

Sugar, as a rule, will add calories with next to zero dietary benefit. The white substance is also known by a few different names, similar to agave, sucrose, high fructose corn syrup, honey, molasses, earthy colored sugar, turbinado, crude sugar, maple syrup, date sugar, malt syrup, hotcake syrup, organic juice condensed, and dextrose.

Recall that 4 to 5 grams of sugar is equivalent to a teaspoon. Experts recommend that most adult women should not consume more than 6 teaspoons (20 grams) a day and adult men 9 teaspoons, or 36 grams. For comparison, a container of pop can have as much as 40 grams, or around 10 teaspoons of sugar.

Nitrates

Sodium nitrate is generally used as a preservative for salty, processed meats like bacon and shop options. Studies have shown that a lot of these ingredients can increase your risk of coronary disease and cancer.

Choose lean, new meats and fish over processed ones however much as could reasonably be expected.

Partially Hydrogenated Oil (Trans Fats)

Trans fats are connected to coronary disease and insulin resistance. Studies have shown that of every dietary fat, trans fats are the most hazardous, especially if you are overweight.

When you see food varieties that say "partially hydrogenated oil," you have discovered as trans fat. Indeed, even food named "0 trans fats" can have up to a portion of a gram. So, it is ideal to know where they hide and stay away from them. The most significant offenders are expected: processed snacks like saltines, chips, and cookies are brimming with them, as are fried food sources and different food varieties utilizing vegetable shortenings and margarine.

Exercising Is A Medication-Free Way To Deal With Bringing Down Hypertension

Poor lifestyle habits, like a lack of exercise, can trigger hypertension. Find how little changes in your day-to-day schedule can have a major effect.

Your risk of hypertension (hypertension) increases with age, however getting some activity can have a major effect. What is more, assuming your blood pressure is now high, exercise can assist you with controlling it. Try not to think you really want to run a long-distance race or join a gym center right away. Instead, begin slow and work more physical activities into your day-to-day routines.

How Exercise Can Bring Down Your Blood Pressure

Regular physical activity or work makes your heart stronger. A stronger heart can circulate more blood with less exertion. Thus, the force on your arteries decreases, bringing down your blood pressure.

Blood pressure is estimated in millimeters of mercury (mm Hg). Ordinary blood pressure is under 120 mm Hg for the top number (systolic) and under 80 mm Hg for the base number (diastolic). Turning out to be more active can bring down both your top and base blood pressure numbers. How much lower is not completely clear, yet research show decreases from 4 to 12 mm Hg diastolic and 3 to 6 mm Hg systolic.

Regular physical activity or exercise can assist you with keeping a healthy weight — one more significant method for controlling blood pressure. In case you are overweight, shedding even 5 pounds (2.3 kilograms) can bring down your blood pressure.

To keep your blood pressure sound, you want to continue to practice consistently. It takes around one to 90 days for regular exercise to affect your blood pressure. The advantages keep going just as long as you keep on working out.

Knowing What Medications To Avoid

Just like you will like to know what kinds of foods to avoid, you will of necessity know what kinds of drugs of medications to avoid.

Some over-the-counter (OTC) drugs can increase your blood pressure while others render your blood pressure medications ineffective. As a high BP sufferer, you need to be wary what OTC drugs to avoid.

Some of the common OTC drugs you need to avoid are as below

Pain-Relivers Such As Non-Steroidal Anti-Inflammatory Drugs (NSAIDs), Like Ibuprofen And Naproxen

NSAIDs include both prescription and over-the-counter drugs. These kinds of medications are often used to alleviate pain or reduce inflammation resulting from conditions like arthritis. NSAIDs can induce your body to retain excess fluid and diminish the functions of your kidneys. This may result in a rise in your blood pressure, exerting more force on your heart and kidneys. This condition, if not reversed or controlled can lead to cardiac arrest or stroke, particularly when this kind of drug was taken in large doses.

Cough and cold drugs, also known as decongestants, especially those that contain pseudoephedrine.

A lot of cough and cold medicines use NSAIDs to relieve pain. As discussed earlier, NSAIDs can increase your blood pressure. Cough and cold drugs usually contain decongestants that can aggravate blood pressure in the following ways. Firstly, decongestants can cause your heart rate and blood pressure to rise. Secondly, decongestants can inhibit the effective working of your blood pressure medication. Finally, pseudoephedrine of sudafed is a special decongestant that have the potential of increasing your blood pressure.

Certain antacids and other stomach drugs that are high in sodium.

Antacids regularly contain decongestants and NSAIDs. Since many of these medicines contain high levels of sodium, they can cause your blood pressure to rise significantly.

Weight Loss Drugs

Certain weight loss medications are known to make heart disease worse. Appetite suppressants tend to boost up your body. This can cause you blood pressure to rise and exert more stress on your heart.

Migraine Headache Drugs

Certain migraine medicines function by constricting the blood vessels in your head. This action helps to alleviate migraine head ache. The problem with this is that they also tighten the blood vessels across your body, leading to your blood pressure rising to unhealthy levels.

If you have high blood pressure or similar type of heart disease, discuss with your doctor before taking a medication.

CHAPTER FIVE

Reversing High Blood Pressure through Physical Exercises:

How much physical exercise do you really need?

You ought to attempt to get somewhere around 150 minutes of moderate aerobic exercise or 75 minutes of rigorous high-impact activity seven days, or a blend of the two. Target at least 30 minutes of vigorous aerobic exercise most days of the week. In the event that you are not used to working out, work gradually toward this objective. You can break your exercise into three 10-minute meetings of high-impact practice and get a similar advantage as one 30-minute program.

Any movement that increases your heart and breathing rates is viewed as aerobic activity, including:

- Dynamic games, like ball or tennis

- Bicycling

- Climbing steps or stairs

- Moving the body or Dancing

- Planting, including trimming the grass and raking leaves

- Running or jogging

- Swimming

- Strolling or walking

A blend of vigorous and weight (resistance) training appears to give the most heart-healthy advantages.

In case you sit for a many hours per day, attempt to enjoy 5-to 10-minute breaks every hour to stretch and move. A non-active (stationary) lifestyle is connected to numerous chronic medical issues, including hypertension. Attempt low-force exercises, for example, going for a speedy stroll or in any event, going to the kitchen or lunchroom to get a drink of water. Setting an update on your telephone or PC might be useful.

When you might require your primary care physician's(doctor') approval

Most times, it is ideal to check with your primary care physician(doctors) before you enroll into an exercise program, especially if:

•   You have a chronic ailment like diabetes, coronary disease or lung sickness.

•   You have elevated cholesterol or hypertension.

•   You've had a coronary failure (or heart attack).

•   You have a family background of heart-related issues before age 55 in men and age 65 in women.

•   You feel pain or distress in your chest, jaw, neck or arms during movement.

•   You become lightheaded with activity.

•   You smoke or as of late stopped smoking.

•   You are overweight or obese.

•   You are uncertain that you are healthy or you have not been exercising routinely.

A few medications, including hypertension drugs, influence your blood pressure and your body's reaction to work out. Likewise, assuming you take blood pressure drugs and as of late increase your activity level, inquire as to whether you want to change your dosage. For certain individuals, getting more activity diminishes their requirement for blood pressure prescription.

Monitor your heart rate

To decrease the risk of injury while working out, begin slowly. Make sure to heat up before you exercise and cool down subsequently. Develop the intensity of your exercises slowly.

Utilize these means to check your pulse (heart rate) during exercise:

• Stop momentarily.

• Gauge your heartbeat for 15 seconds. To examine your heartbeat over your carotid artery, put your first and third fingers on your neck to the side of your windpipe. To actually look at your heartbeat at your wrist, place two fingers between the bone and the ligament over your radial artery — which is situated on the thumb side of your wrist.

• Multiply this number by 4 to ascertain your heart beats per minute.

Here is a model: You quit exercising and gauge your heartbeat for 15 seconds, getting 37 pulses. Multiply 37 by 4, to get 148 beats per minute.

Quit Exercising When You feel pain

Quit exercising and look for immediate medical attention in the event that you have any advance indications of impending heart issues during exercise, including:

• Chest, neck, jaw or arm pain or snugness

• Dazedness or faintness

• Extreme windedness or difficulty breathing

• An unpredictable heartbeat (irregular heart pulse)

Track Your Progress

The best way to recognize and monitor hypertension is to monitor your blood pressure readings. Have your blood pressure checked at each specialist's visit and utilize a home blood pressure monitor. While checking your blood pressure at home, it is ideal to do as such regularly at the same periods every day.

The best activities to control hypertension

Do you need to drop your blood pressure by up to 20 points? Probably the most effective way to achieve this is by getting back to your ideal body weight. You can ascertain it by deciding your body mass index (BMI).

To help you achieve your weight objective, and to assist with bringing down your blood pressure meanwhile, think about these six activities or exercises, says a specialist cardiologist.

Ten minutes of brisk or moderate strolling three times each day

Exercise brings down blood pressure by reducing blood vessel firmness so blood can stream all the more without any problem. The impacts of activity are generally noticeable during and following an exercise. Reduced blood pressure can be most significant just after you work out.

Along these lines, wellbeing experts recommend, the best method for combatting hypertension may be to break your exercise into a few sessions over the course of the day. Truth be told, one investigation discovered that three 10-minute strolls a day more really forestalled future blood pressure spikes than one 30-minute journey each day.

Thirty minutes per day of trekking or fixed cycling, or three 10-minute squares of cycling

Similar thinking applies here as it applies for strolling.

Climbing or Hiking

The muscle power expected to ascend a street on a grade, a slope or a mountain can assist you with accomplishing a more prominent degree of wellness. Actual work, for example, climbing can bring down blood pressure up to 10 points.

Work area treadmilling or pedal pushing

BP readings were much more ideal in a review where participants strolled along at a sluggish 1-mile-per-hour pace at work area-based treadmills for no less than 10 minutes consistently, or accelerated exercise bikes under a work area for somewhere around 10 minutes consistently.

Power lifting

Despite the fact that it sounds counter-intuitive, weight lifting or lifting can lessen blood pressure. Strength training really raises blood pressure levels for a brief time, however can assist by and large wellness, which will further improve blood pressure levels also.

Swimming

This type of activity can be gainful in controlling blood pressure in adults of 60 years and older, another study has found. Over a duration of 12 weeks, swimming participants slowly moved as long as 45 minutes of constant swimming at a time. By the end of the review, the swimmers had decreased their systolic blood pressure by an average of nine points.

Authorities on the subject matter believe that the advantages of exercise are not realized in the event that the exercise is not sustained. Expert specialists also trust that the 'put it to work, or it will stop' hypothesis is valid. You can lose gains in the wake of halting exercise for a long time. Moderate exercise for 150 minutes of the week or rigorous exercise for 75 minutes of the week is the standard recommendation.

CHAPTER SIX

Could lack of sleep be a cause of hypertension?

Perhaps. Sleep specialists prescribe that adult ought to get seven to eight hours of a sleep every night. Getting under six hours of sleep is known to be terrible for your general wellbeing. Stress, jet lag, shift duties and other sleep disturbances make you susceptible to coronary diseases and increase the risk for heart diseases, including obesity and diabetes. A regular absence of sleep might prompt high blood pressure (hypertension) in both children and adults.

The less you sleep, the higher your blood pressure might go. Individuals who sleep six hours or less may have more extreme increases in blood pressure. On the likelihood that you as of now have hypertension, not sleeping soundly may aggravate your blood pressure.

It is believed that sleep assists your body with controlling hormones expected to manage blood pressure and digestion (or metabolism). Over the long periods, an absence of sleep could cause swings in hormones, triggering hypertension and other risk factors for coronary diseases.

Try not to attempt to compensate for an absence of sleep with a great deal of sleep. An excessive amount of sleep, less significantly than short rest, can trigger high sugar and weight gain, which are bad for your heart wellbeing. Discuss with your PCP (primary-care physician) for tips on getting better sleep, particularly if you have hypertension.

One potential, treatable cause for your absence of sleep contributing to hypertension is obstructive sleep apnea — a sleep problem where you constantly pause and begin breathing during sleep. Discuss with your primary care physician in the event that you feel tired even following an entire night's sleep, especially if you wheeze or snore. Obstructive sleep apnea might be the reason. Obstructive sleep apnea can increase your risk of hypertension and other heart-related issues.

Getting More Sleep Can Ease Hypertension

As reported by the CDC, around one of every three Americans are said to have hypertension, a statistic that has increased gradually throughout recent years and makes it clear that things are not pulling back. Ranging from heritage or legacy, a bad eating routine and an absence of sleep, more individuals are experiencing hypertension than any time in recent memory.

Most Americans likewise gripe about being sleepless, a CDC statistic that has additionally been rising as of late. Both an absence of sleep and high blood pressure, otherwise called hypertension, can influence each other fundamentally and ought to be attended to with urgency. We will go over what hypertension is, what an absence of sleep can mean for it, and how you might get to bed and lower your blood pressure.

How Hypertension is Impacted by Sleep

There is a reasonable linkage between how much sleep somebody gets and their risk of hypertension. In a new report on the connection between sleep duration and the risk of hypertension, specialists found the individuals who sleep under 4 hours a night were at a lot more susceptible than the people who sleep 7 hours every night.

Nonetheless, this investigation likewise discovered that sleeping too lengthy can likewise build your risk of hypertension — this issue can be avoided by getting the recommended amount of sleep every single night, which differs from one individual to another.

In another review, scientists observed that individuals who just slept six hours the earlier night are displayed to have worse hypertension the following day when contrasted with the people who had an extraordinary night's sleep. Protracted absence of sleep can intensify this impact. Without adequate sleep to revitalize your body, you could be stressing on yourself without acknowledging it until it is past the point of no return.

A clinical therapist believes that hypertension is a key cardiovascular risk factor. There are currently many examinations that have had the option to show that deficient sleep and poor sleep quality are connected with the advancement of hypertension and different parts of coronary diseases.

If you already suffer from the symptoms of sleep apnea, having hypertension can be an additional burden. Sleep apnea is caused, ordinarily, by the rear of the throat unwinding and constricting oxygen flow or stream into the body. Those experiencing sleep apnea are more at risk of having hypertension.

While experiencing hypertension and sleep apnea together, oxygen circulating through the body is incredibly decreased. Sleep apnea can increase blood pressure by decreasing oxygen that you are taking. The higher your blood pressure climbs, the more in danger you are having medical issues like congestive cardiovascular breakdown and stroke.

Instructions on How to Control Hypertension with Sleep

There is good news on if you are currently battling with hypertension. Symptoms can be captured quickly with regular physicals. The treatment for hypertension can be managed. Simple adjustments like to slimming down, exercising and sleeping regimens can have an immense effect in your life.

In the event that you have a background marked by hypertension in your family, it is smart to stay aware of standard checkups on the grounds that hypertension is genetic. Catching it early will reduce your risk of greater issues down the line.

While diet and exercise are critical to treating hypertension, sleep is an everyday routine that most disregard in their treatment plan. By changing how you sleep and what you sleep on, you can significantly decrease your blood pressure.

Pick a Comfortable Mattress or Sleeping pad

Assuming you feel languid and in pain in the morning, it very well might be an indication that the time has come to overhaul your sleeping cushion. Traditional innerspring beddings or mattresses commonly begin turning out to be less comfortable around the eighth year of use. It is possible that throughout that period of time, you may be sleeping poorly and not being conscious of it since you have become acclimated with how you are sleeping now.

Pick the best bedding for your sleeping style to ensure you are essentially as comfortable as possible as you sleep. Less thrashing or tossing around at midnight implies additional time getting great, serene sleep. Your body will rejuvenate from the day activity and stress as well as allow you to sleep longer during that time without interference.

Pursue Sound Sleeping Routines

Other than changing what you sleep on, you ought to likewise change how you view sleep to battle hypertension all the more successfully. This will include how you approach your nights and what to do once you are sleeping.

Before you get into bed, there is a great deal that should be possible to make your nights more effective. Having a lighter supper prior in the day will permit your body to process the food and stay away from awkward indigestion.

In the hour leading up to bedtime, leave your gadgets or devices like mobile phones or PCs to slow down. Blue light produced from these screens sets off your minds to remain alert since this light emulates daylight. Unwinding with a book, a warm shower, or another evening custom will tell your brain that it is sleep time.

When you are in bed, you ought to zero in on sleeping to assist with reinforcing the relationship in your brain between your bed and getting drained. Doing this consistently can assist with making it more straightforward to nod off rather than marathon watching television or looking at web-based entertainment or social media.

Be Benevolent to Your Body

Being sleepless makes the day harder than it should be. A protracted absence of sleep can have significant ramifications for your wellbeing, including hypertension. Hypertension can be managed, yet provided that you roll out the right improvements in your day-to-day lifestyle.

As indicated by a prestigious specialist, sound sleep is progressively becoming perceived as a significant piece of generally wellbeing and health. Studies are demonstrating the way that further developing sleep can decrease the risks of hypertension and other cardiovascular maladies.

Begin by treating your body well and focusing on sleep to assist with battling the risk of hypertension. Utilizing breathable, cotton sheets will likewise give you an oxygen support and increase blood flow to assist with keeping you healthy as you sleep. This will permit your body to unwind around evening time and spotlight exclusively on the act of dozing.

What Is The Best Sleeping Position?

The best sleeping position is certainly not a one-size-fits-all. Individuals sleep in different ways. Every individual has different necessities and is comfortable in varying sleeping position. Think about something beyond comfort to track down the best sleeping position for you. Different sleeping positions have different advantages. Assuming you are currently battling with pain or other medical issues, you could have to change your sleeping position to manage it. Also, while it may not be something you can do in one night, it could merit an attempt.

Creating the opportunity to steadily prepare yourself to sleep in another position could be secret to working on the quality of your sleep. Nevertheless, in case this is something you are not happy with, do not stress over it. You can also attempt to change your favorite rest position to ensure you capitalize on it. Everyone is unique. What is important is that you do what works for your body and the sleep you require. Poor sleeping conditions might actually be the fundamental reason for lower back ache. This is because a few positions can put undue strain on the neck, hips, and back.

Different Sleeping Positions

Sleeping on The Back with Knee Support
Lying on the back is well known to be the best sleeping position for a healthy back. This position distributes the weight to the full length of the body most significant surface. It likewise limits pressure points and guarantees adequate arrangement of the head, neck, and spine. Putting a little pad under the knees will offer additional help and assist with keeping up with the regular bend of the spine.

Sleeping on the Side with A Pillow in Between The Knees
Despite the fact that lying on the side is a well-known and pleasant sleeping position, the spine can be skewed out of position. This could strain the lower back. Fixing this is simple. Anybody who sleeps on their side can simply put a firm cushion or pillow between their knees. This raises the upper leg, reestablishing the normal arrangement of the hips, pelvis, and spine.

Sleeping in The Crouch Position

For people with herniated disks, taking a twisted fetal position might bring relief during the night. That is because lying on the side with the knees in the chest decreases the twisting of the spine and assists with opening up the joints.

Sleeping on The Front with a Cushion Under the Stomach

Lying before the body is for the most part viewed as the most awful sleeping position. Notwithstanding, for those battling to sleep in another position, putting a thin pad or pillow under the stomach and hips can assist with working on the alignment of the spine. Sleeping on the front may likewise help individuals with herniated plate disease or degenerative disk disease.

Sleeping On the Anterior with The Head Face Down

One more explanation that sleeping on the front is viewed as awful as the head is turned on one side only. This turns the spine and puts extra weight on the neck, shoulders, and back. Make an attempt at lying face down to avoid this. A little but firm pillow or even a firmly rolled towel can be used to set up the forehead, creating allowance to breathe properly. This should be done alongside the use of a pad or pillow under the stomach.

Sleeping On the Back in A Leaned-back Position

Sleeping in a leaned-back position might help lower back pain, particularly in individuals with isthmic spondylolisthesis. If significant huge help is found from resting in a reclined back seat, it could be wise to put invest into a customizable bed which can be adjusted in like manner.

Sleeping Hygiene

Back pain can cause critical sleep disturbances. People should endeavor not to sleep late to make up for overnight sleep loss. Everything being equal, they ought to attempt to keep a standard timetable consistent with sleep time and wake-up times. Most adults need somewhere in the range of 7 and 9 hours per night. Some vital sleep hygiene tips include:

o   Avoiding energizers, like caffeine, around evening time

o   Trying to keep away from intense exercises in the hours leading up to sleep time

o   Winding down before genuine sleep time by reading, taking a warm bath, listening to soothing music, or doing a light yoga session

o   Make the room relaxing by darkening the lights and eliminating interruptions, like PCs, mobile phones and televisions.

Best Sleeping Position During Pregnancy

Lying down on one side is prescribed as the best posture to sleep during pregnancy. Research demonstrates that from 20 weeks into pregnancy, the left side position can significantly improve the progression of blood to the baby. Most women report spending of time sleeping on the back during pregnancy, yet this position is not recommended as it very high likelihood of resulting to stillbirth following 28 weeks of pregnancy. The greater part of the studies emphasized on the increased need of sleep during pregnancy. The elevated degrees of hormones expected to keep up with pregnancy likewise causes sleepiness. Simultaneously, it is exceptionally normal for pregnant women to suffer back pain, acid reflux, queasiness, and extreme night urination, all of which might interfere with sleep. In addition to these, pregnancy increases the risk of sleep disorders, for example, obstructive sleep disorders.

CHAPTER SEVEN

Monitor Your Body Mass Index

Body Mass Index (BMI) is a measurement of an individual weight in comparison to his or her height. It is a more of a pointer than an accurate measurement of an individual's body fat. BMI, as a rule, correlates well with total body fat. This shows that as the BMI score increases, so does an individual's complete body fat.

The WHO classifies an adult who has a BMI somewhere in the range of 25 and 29.9 as overweight - an adult who has a BMI of 30 or higher considered obese - a BMI below 18.5 is viewed as underweight, and between 18.5 to 24.9 a healthy weight.

The most effective method to gauge your BMI (How To Measure Your BMI)

BMI in an individual is determined by the use of a numerical formula. It can likewise be evaluated in tables in which one can match height in inches to weight in pounds to estimate BMI. There are accessible calculators online that can help one calculate his or her BMI index.

The equation is - BMI = (Weight in kilograms) divided by (Height in meters squared)

A normal BMI index is one that falls somewhere in the range of 18.5 and 24.9. This shows that an individual is within the typical weight territory for their height. A BMI graph is used to classify an individual as underweight, normal, overweight, or obese.BMI is a measure of total fat in many people. Hence it is considered as a pointer of health risk.BMI is utilized by medical services experts to screen for overweight and obese people. The BMI is used to evaluate an individual's health risk in relation to with obesity and overweight.

For instance, those with a high BMI are in danger of:

- high blood cholesterol or other lipid disorders

- type 2 diabetes

- coronary (or heart) disease

- stroke

- hypertension

- certain tumors (or cancers)

- gallbladder disease

- sleep apnea and wheezing(snoring)

- untimely death

- osteoarthritis and joint disease

- For a significant amount of people, BMI can be utilized to give a decent indication of obesity. However, BMI does not to give real data on body constitution like measure of muscle, bone, fat, and different tissues.

- In certain people BMI is a more exact proportion of fat than others. For instance, people who are very muscular might fall into the overweight category when they are really sound and exceptionally fit. These people with an exceptionally low muscle versus fat ratio could have similar BMI score as somebody who is overweight.

- Likewise, an older and fragile individual might be in the normal weight class or category when they have little muscle and a high level of body fat.

- BMI, when utilized for kids and adolescents who are as yet developing, those with huge body frames or modest forms, pregnant women and profoundly ripped people in this manner should be evaluate and interpreted meticulously.

Monitor Your Blood Pressure Regularly

To gauge blood pressure, your doctor utilizes an instrument call a sphygmomanometer, which mostly known as a blood pressure cuff. The cuff is folded over your upper arm and expanded to stop the progression of blood in your artery. As the cuff is gradually collapsed, your doctor utilizes a stethoscope to listen to the blood flowing through the artery. These beating sounds register on a measure joined to the cuff. The first pumping sound your doctor hears is recorded as the systolic pressure, and the last strong is the diastolic pressure.

Be that as it may, today there are loads of programmed or digital sphygmomanometers which you can purchase of Amazon or any drug store. You really want to keep one at home with the goal that you can routinely screen your blood pressure levels at home.

How to monitor Blood Pressure by Yourself

DIY testing

There are two conditions in which you could check your blood pressure at home. One is on the grounds that your doctor has asked you to, or on the grounds that you need to watch out for it yourself. Assuming that you are taking medicine or making life style changes to reduce your blood pressure, it can assist you with laying out objectives and monitor your progress. The reality is that patients who check their own blood pressure by themselves regularly at home are bound to find lasting success in their goals.

Also, assuming that you are one of those individuals whose blood pressure goes up whenever you visit a specialist, a medical procedure or clinic lounge area (this condition is known as white-coat hypertension), scanning it at home can give a more realistic picture of what it resembles in addition to being in casual everyday circumstances.

How does a blood pressure monitor work?

Blood pressure is gauged by using a sphygmomanometer, or blood pressure monitor. It comprises of an inflatable sleeve or cuff that is folded over your arm, generally to level with your heart, and a checking gadget that actions the sleeve's tension.

The reading estimates two pressures: systolic, and diastolic. Systolic pressure is higher, occurring when your heart beats and pushes blood through the arteries, and diastolic pressure is estimated when your heart is resting and filling up with blood. In this way, for instance, your blood pressure may be 120 over 80.

Blood pressure reading can be manual or computerized or digital, yet home monitoring is generally digital and the entire estimation process is programmed aside from putting the cuff around your arm.

The sleeve then expands until it fits firmly around your arm, cutting off your blood stream, and afterward the valve opens to collapse it. As the sleeve arrives at your systolic strain, blood starts to stream around your artery. This makes a vibration that is identified by the meter, which records your systolic strain. In a conventional simple sphygmomanometer, the blood sounds are recognized by the specialist utilizing a stethoscope.

As the sleeve keeps on flattening, it arrives at your diastolic pressure, and the vibration stops. The meter detects this, and records the pressure once more.

How to take BP readings?

Taking readings requires some thought and planning, however before long, it will turn out to be natural. There is a few things to remember:

•	Loosen up. Avoid caffeine and exercise for thirty minutes ahead of time, and rest for a couple of minutes. Sit in a relaxed upright position with your feet level on the floor and with your back straight up.

•	Position your arm accurately. Lay it on a level surface, with your upper arm level with your heart.

•	Position the sleeve or cuff accurately, with the base edge simply over your elbow.

The guidance manual of your gadget or device will likewise give you clear guidelines or instructions.

When to check blood pressure?

Assuming that you're utilizing a blood pressure monitor on your doctor's recommendation, then he or she should let you know when to take readings. When in doubt, however, you ought to check them during similar periods of day on each event, so you're comparing like and with like.

Take a couple of readings each time, two or three minutes apart, and calculate the average to make the figures more representative. Furthermore, in the event that your blood pressure monitor doesn't store your readings for you, write them down in a note pad to find out about long-term patterns.

CHAPTER EIGHT

Conclusion

Turning around hypertension is truly achievable by following a routine of carrying on with a healthy lifestyle as well as following a DASH diet, including habitual exercise and following a sound sleep design. Hypertension is seen to be majorly a lifestyle disease, and in my view. 50% of high blood pressure cases result from unhealthy life style choices, while 25% is caused by genetic factors or hereditary predisposition and the last 25% can be attributable to secondary causes such as underlying diseases like CKD (chronic kidney disease) and the like.

You can significantly reduce your high blood pressure over a 90-day period by adjusting your lifestyle, dietary habits and sleep. Get more active, watch what you eat and ensure you get at least 6 to 7 hours of sleep every night. Keep monitoring and checking your BP and BMI numbers to keep track of and sustain progress on a daily, weekly and monthly basis.

* 9 7 9 8 3 4 4 8 7 9 9 0 1 *